Dash Diet

Discover Delicious And Nutritious Low-Sodium Recipes For Blood Pressure Reduction With A 30-day Meal Plan

(Reduce Your Weight And Take Charge Of Your Health)

Gabriel Haywood

TABLE OF CONTENT

Introduction – What Is Dash?

An estimated 70 million Americans, or nearly one in three adults, suffer from hypertension, according to estimates. Hypertension is not only a risk for adults; children are also susceptible. The American diet is loaded with dietary sources that increase pulse rate. Hypertension can increase the risk for a variety of other medical conditions, including stroke and heart disease. DASH is an acronym for Dietary Approaches to Prevent Hypertension. The DASH regimen was designed to reduce circulatory strain without medication. Studies indicate that it can reduce the risk of hypertension-related illnesses and perplexity. Since its inception in the 2 990s, the original eating routine has been modified and transformed into a dual-purpose diet.

It was conceived by clinical specialists, researchers, and nutritionists, and was based solely on research without any corporate funding. The DASH diet is based on a determination of investigation that goes beyond simply reducing sodium intake. It is a diet that emphasizes whole foods, low-fat dairy, and whole cereals and has been shown to be significantly more effective than low sodium alone. Several public organizations, including the American Heart Association and the National Heart, Lung, and Blood Institute, recommend this diet. Even the ADA has praised it as a "excellent way for

Americans to eat." Results indicate that this regimen is equally effective for children (since even children can develop hypertension!).

It is recommended as an example of a healthy diet that anyone, regardless of hypertension, can follow. In fact, observing the DASH diet if you are at risk for hypertension can help prevent you from developing it.

The DASH diet works by supplying the body with specific nutrients in greater quantities and restricting those that raise heart rate. The most popular hypertension calorie counting diet restricts sodium to 26 00mg, whereas the DASH diet restricts it to 2 10 00mg and focuses on food varieties rich in Magnesium, Calcium, and Potassium, which are incredibly important for lowering pulse. Despite this restriction, the diet is extremely straightforward to adhere to.

Many individuals who adhere to the DASH diet experience additional benefits, the most well-known of which is weight loss. However, others have reported that they look and feel younger and have experienced improved outcomes in other clinical conditions, such as diabetes. The Dietary Approaches to Stop Hypertension (DASH) diet focuses on a whole-foods diet and additional lifestyle changes that teach individuals how to live a generally healthier lifestyle, not just consume better. This fashion consumes fewer calories than the majority of current trends because it can be adapted to suit the needs of any individual. This is why it is so effective.

It appears simple, but something so captivating must have a secret ingredient, right?

The relationship between Sodium and Blood Pressure

Some individuals are at a greater risk for hypertension than others. Those who are obese, older than sixty, or African American are particularly at risk. A diet heavy in sodium causes the body to retain water. The sodium in the salt acts as a sort of magnet for water and absorbs it. If you consider reconstituted food varieties, they are frequently salted to remove moisture and preserve the food. In the same way, your body absorbs salt into its cells, which then swell with water. The abundance of liquids makes it more difficult for the heart to syphon blood, thereby increasing heart rate. By decreasing sodium, the body is no longer managing an excess of fluid and the heart can pump more efficiently.

Blood pressure is the force exerted by the blood against supply route barriers. The presence of hypertension signifies that this parameter is greater than average. The number will fluctuate throughout the day depending on what you eat and what you do. For instance, our resting and awakening pulses are lower than our running pulses. Regardless, how does this translate into the statistics we see when hypertension is discussed?

The values are separated into systolic and diastolic components. The systolic number represents the strain when the heart is beating, whereas the diastolic number gauges the time between heartbeats. The amount is estimated using mercury millimeters. The standard ratio is 2 20/80ml. At this time, it is not entirely clear what causes these numbers. Several factors, such as aging, weight, hereditary characteristics, and nutrition, have been cited as contributors to the rise in obesity, but only diet is one that we can actually influence. This is why the DASH method is so important. We can treat hypertension twice as effectively by utilizing the DASH diet and possibly taking prescription medication to additionally circumvent our hereditary characteristics. With a healthy diet and regular exercise, medication becomes unnecessary.

Why 2 8 Days?

The initial DASH plan has no time limit. Dietary Approach to Stopping Hypertension and Hyperlipidemia (DASH) is a fourteen-day weight loss plan. The difference between the two is that while the original DASH focuses solely on lowering blood pressure, the weight loss version is also designed to aid in weight loss. The two phases each last fourteen days, and they can be cycled; however, once you've reached stage two, it's best to stick with it, as a relapse can cause your blood pressure to rise. The stages consist of the following:

Phase One: During this time, you are expected to learn how to eat properly and which foods stimulate digestion for weight loss. The first fourteen days are dedicated to ensuring that you are not hungry and are consuming nutritious meals. Stage one is by far the most difficult because you are attempting to remove a large number of items and then reintroduce them later. You must avoid dull food sources, such as breads and processed sugars, and choose sources of protein and fiber. Additionally, it is prudent to avoid alcoholic beverages because they are rich in regular sugar. Dairy is permissible so long as it is low in fat, but you should limit your consumption of cheddar due to the high sodium content of most processed cheeses. You're avoiding bland foods and sugar because they will cause your blood sugar to spike and then collapse, resulting in cravings for another high. By avoiding them for the first fourteen days, you will have fewer cravings and greater glucose control. Most whole vegetables are straightforward replacements for bland snack options and are more effective at preventing blood sugar spikes. During stage one, you should concentrate on consuming four to five servings of beans or lentils per week for their protein and fiber content. You'll also need to limit yourself to 6 ounces of fish or lean meat per day, which is significantly less than what the majority of us consume. Solid lipids, such as nuts and seeds, are recommended, but you must also avoid fruits and vegetables due to their high sugar content.

Phase Two: After completing the foundational phase, you can gradually reintroduce certain food types to your diet. In general, stage two is the maintenance portion of your diet, as it must be adhered to indefinitely to maintain a healthy weight and heart rate. You can reintroduce 6 to 8 daily servings of whole grains, 8 to 10 daily servings of natural product, 6 weekly servings of sugar, and swap one daily serving of natural product for one glass of wine.

The difference between this diet and the first DASH option is that there is a greater emphasis on whole grain food sources during the maintenance phase.

Certain nutrition types are eradicated permanently by numerous extreme weight control plans, which makes them so difficult to adhere to. Instead of prohibiting popular foods like pasta and bread, the DASH diet permits you to consume them with moderation and in a more nutritious form. With this small adjustment, you should not encounter any problems for the rest of your life. In a perfect world, you would need to divide your food intake into six small meals throughout the day, as opposed to three large meals, to prevent excessive snacking and blood sugar surges.

Chapter 1: The Foods To Avoid For The Brain Diet

The MIND diet recommends limiting these five foods:

Butter and margarine: Tru consumes less than 2 tableroon (approximately 2 8 grams) of dalu. Instead, use olive oil as your cooking fat and drizzle your bread with olive oil and herbs.

CHEESE: The MIND diet recommends limiting your sleep duration to no more than one week.

NO MORE THAN THREE SERVINGS OF RED MEAT PER WEEK. This includes all beef, pork, lamb, and meat products containing these meats.

FRIED FOOD: The MIND diet discourages cold foods, especially those from fast-food restaurants. Limit your son's visit to no more than once per week.

PASTRIES AND SWEETS: These include the majority of the sugary snack foods and desserts that come to mind. Ise sream, sookies, brownies, snask sakes, donuts, sandu and more. Truly limit yourselves to no more than four times per week. Researchers recommend limiting consumption of these foods because they contain saturated and trans fats. Trans fats are clearly associated with all types of maladies, including heart disease and Alzheimer's disease, according to research. However, the health effects of saturated fat are hotly contested in the field of nutrition. Although the research on saturated fat and heart disease may be flawed and highly suspect, animal research and human observational studies suggest that consuming saturated fat in excess is linked to poor mental health. The MIND Diet Reduces oxidative stress and inflammation. Current research on the MIND det has not been able to determine "exactly how it operates." However, the individuals who designed the diet believe it will be effective by reducing oxidative stress and inflammation. Oxidative stress occurs when significant quantities of unstable molecules and free radicals accumulate in the body. This often sauses damage to sells. The bran is particularly susceptible to the nature of damage.

Our body's natural response to injury and infection is inflammation. However, if not properly regulated, inflammability can also be harmful and contribute to human disease.Oxidative stress and inflammation can be extremely detrimental to the brain. Recent years have seen the development of interventions to prevent and treat Alzheimer's disease. Following the Mediterranean and DASH diets is associated with reduced oxidative stress and inflammation. Because the MIND diet is a combination of these two diets, the foods that contribute to a healthy MIND diet also have anti-oxidant and anti-inflammatory properties. The anti-oxidant in blueberries and the vitamin E Olive oil, green leafy vegetables, and nuts are believed to improve brain function by protecting it from oxidative stress.In addition, the omega-6 fatty acids found in fish are well-known for their ability to reduce inflammation in the brain and have been linked to reduced cognitive function loss.

Chapter 2: The Mind Diet May Reduce Harmful Beta-Amyloid Proteins

Researchers also believe that the MIND diet can benefit the brain by reducing the detrimental beta-amyloid beta-amyloid.

Beta-amulod rroten are fragments of rroten found naturally in the body. However, they can assume and form plaques that build up in the brain, impairing communication between brain cells and resulting in the death of brain cells. Many people believe that these rlaues are among the rrmaru saues of Alzheimer's disease. Anmal and test-tube tude ugge that the antoxdant and micronutrients found in MIND det food may aid in preventing the formation of beta-amyloid plaques in the brain. In addition, the MIND diet restricts foods containing saturated and trans fats, which studies have shown can increase beta-amyloid receptor protein levels in the brain. Human observational studies have shown that consuming these fats is associated with a doubling of the risk of developing Alzheimer's disease. Nonetheless, it is essential to note that the nature of research cannot determine cause and effect. Higher-quality, randomized studies are required to determine precisely how the MIND diet can promote brain health.

Chapter 3: Dietary Methods To Prevent Hypertension

This diet was originally devised in 2 992 as a means of reducing the prevalence of morbid hypertension among Americans. Today, after years of exhaustive research by various health institutions, the United States government promotes the DASH diet not only for individuals with hypertension, but also as a healthy model diet for all Americans to prevent chronic diseases.

The DASH (Dietary Approaches to Stop Hypertension) diet encourages increased fruit, vegetable, whole grain, and low-fat dairy rrodust consumption. The diet also calls for lean meat, fish, quinoa, nuts, and beans as alternative sources of protein and advises a general reduction in sodium, sugar, and fat. Maximum daily salt consumption was 6 ,200 mg from all sources. The maximum amount of sugar allowed was three tearoon onlu. Alsohol consumption is restricted to a maximum of two beverages per day, and consumption of caffeinated beverages such as coffee and soda is limited to three beverages per day.

Although not entirely vegetarian, the DASH diet can reduce blood pressure by 6 mm Hg in the systolic and 6 mm Hg in the diastolic in individuals with normal blood pressure. Individuals with hypertension experience a decline of 2 2 mm Hg and a 6 mm Hg rerestivelu. This is a substantial reduction and substantial gain for preventing further arterial hardening, heart failure, kidney disease, and coronary heart disease. It applied to men and women between the ages of 8 8 and 86 .

This diet is simple to follow, but be wary of foods labeled "healthy" that conceal significant amounts of sodium, white sugar, and fats. See the labeling for sodium rehydration salt, sugar alcohols, and saturated lipids. DASH diet maintains ideal body weight, which is superior to novelty diets that cause extreme weight loss.

Dietary Arrroashe to Stor Hurertenion (DASH) is a rhuian-recommended, researched, and utilized diet to lower blood pressure in two weeks.

Today, one in four Americans (approximately 76 million people) have hypertension or elevated blood pressure. Blood flow is determined by the pressure within the arterial walls. Hypertension can be defined as a persistent increase in blood pressure. The leading cause of heart attack and stroke, high blood pressure causes the heart to work harder. Reducing your sodium intake and eating a healthy diet can help you reduce your risk of hypertension. This is the DASH diet's premise.

Two studies were conducted by the National Heart, Lung, and Blood Institute regarding this diet. Blood pressure was reduced by consuming a diet low in saturated fat, cholesterol, and total fat and high in fruits, vegetables, fat-free milk, whole grains, fish, rooltru, and almonds.

As you can see, this diet permits a greater variety of foods than other commercially available diets. In addition, you should reduce, but not eliminate, your intake of lean red meat, sweets, added carbohydrates, and sugar-containing beverages. Foodies will not have a difficult time adapting to this diet, as it does not essentially eliminate common American foods.

Recipes and dietary recommendations are provided in the DASH Diet plan for a 2,6 00 mg and 2 ,10 00 mg sodium intake. Approximately 2,6 00 mg of sodium is recommended by both the National High Blood Pressure Education Program and the Dietary Guidelines for Americans. And unlike most short-term diet plans, the

DASH diet also provides guidance on how to stick to the diet. ponder the long term. Although weight loss is not a rrioritu, it is a welcome side effect of the DASH diet, which is predicated on a 2,000-calorie-per-day caloric restriction. Some tips for further reducing sodium in the diet include:

Consult food labels. You will be astonished by how much sodium is present in low-fat and reduced-calorie foods.

No excess salt, rlease. It is customary to add a pinch of salt when steaming rice or bread. Discover alternative spices or botanicals to replace the salt in your standard recipes. A teaspoon of table salt contains 2,6 00 milligrams of sodium.

It is also preferable to make this change gradually, as detoxification reactions such as loss of appetite may prevent you from implementing this diet strategy. Adding some physical activity and receiving appropriate medical care are also advantageous.

In summation, there are a great deal of nutritious but unappealing foods on the market today. The DASH diet allows for ample leg room, and its long-term benefit is a healthier, extended life.

Why not incorporate some DASH into your diet today?

Chapter 4: Benefits Of Dash Diet

You will consume more nutritious meals.

This will require some adjustment, especially for those who have never spent much time in the kitchen. You will be able to enjoy significantly more scrumptious, nutrient-dense meals due to the increased consumption of fresh produce and decreased consumption of processed food.

Spend some time trying new fruits and vegetables and experimenting with various salt-free seasonings in order to create a healthy meal that suits your taste and that your family will enjoy. Instead of grabbing an uisk andwish or fast food burger, a little planning and a focus on the DASH diet will result in the consumption of significantly more nutritious food.

You will reduce your blood pressure.

Obviously, this is the greatest advantage of following the DASH diet, as it is designed specifically to achieve this objective. This diet is a great option for those who are currently taking medication to control their blood pressure or who wish to better manage the symptoms of prehypertension.

You will have healthier levels of cholesterol.

Dietary fiber from fruits and vegetables, whole grains, nuts, and beans, along with lean cuts of meat and fish, and a restricted intake of desserts and refined carbohydrates, have been shown to reduce cholesterol levels. Even with a higher fat version of the diet, which also increases "good" cholesterol, this improvement persists.

You will reduce your risk of developing osteoporosis.

Most dietary "strategies" for the prevention and treatment of osteoporosis involve an increase in vitamin D and calcium consumption, both of which are abundant in many of the foods included in the DASH diet. In addition, research has shown that reducing sodium intake can be an effective treatment, proving that the DASH diet can improve bone health.

Following the DASH diet resulted in "significantly increased bone turnover," which, if maintained over an extended period of time, may eventually improve bone mineral density. Additionally, the diet is rich in magneium, vitamin C, antioxidants, and rolurhenol, all of which have been positively associated with enhanced bone health.

You will experience optimal weight maintenance.

Whether you're trying to lose weight or not, the DASH diet is an excellent way to ensure you reach and maintain your ideal weight. You can follow a customized version of the DASH diet to accomplish your weight loss goals, then increase your calorie intake to maintain your new weight. Thanks to the healthy foods included in this diet, you won't have to worry about regaining weight after working so hard to shed pounds.

The DASH diet provides ample protein without excessive carbohydrates, so you can build muscle and increase your metabolism without ever feeling weighed down. This is not a temporary diet; this is a new, healthy lifestyle.

6. With it, you will be able to tisk.

Because this diet is composed of readily available, delectable foods, it is much simpler to adhere to. Once you've committed to the DASH diet, you'll be able to experience a permanent lifestyle change that will have a significant positive impact on your overall health and wellness.

The DASH diet is even simple to follow when dining out; you just need to be aware of which foods will sabotage your efforts. There are numerous ways to make the DASH diet work for you, which is an enormous benefit for anyone seeking to improve their health.

Your kidneys will be in better health.

This diet has been shown to reduce the risk of developing kidney disease and kidney stones, thanks to the potassium, magnesium, fiber, and calcium found in the DASH-approved foods. The diet's emphasis on sodium restriction is also recommended for those at risk for developing kidney disease.

However, the diet should not be followed by individuals who have already been diagnosed with kidney disease or who are undergoing dialysis without the supervision of a health care professional, as it may result in severe side effects.

8 You will be more resistant to certain malignancies.

Researchers have examined the relationship between the DASH diet and different types of cancer and have discovered a positive association between reducing sodium intake and monitoring dietary fat consumption. The diet is also low in red meat, which has been linked to colon, rectal, esophagus, stomach, lung, bronchus, and kidney cancer.

The emphasis on fresh produce helps prevent a number of colon cancers, while the emphasis on low-fat dairy products contributes to a diminished risk of colon cancer.

You will have the ability to prevent diabetes.

The DASH diet has been shown to be effective in preventing insulin resistance, which has been linked to elevated blood pressure and sardiovasular health risks. By helping dieters control their sodium intake, consume more fiber and potassium, and maintain a healthy weight, the DASH eating plan helps those who are predisposed to develop diabetes or delay its onset.

According to a number of studies, this effect is amplified when the DASH diet is incorporated into a comprehensive health regimen that includes diet, exercise, and weight control.

2 0. You'll avoid feeling famished.

Thanks to a high intake of fiber and protein, the DASH diet will never leave its adherents with unhealthy food cravings; rather, you will feel satiated throughout the day and look forward to your next nutritious, substantial meal. Nonetheless, it's a good idea to plan ahead so you can bring DASH-approved snacks just in case.

Low-fat and calorie-restricted diets can leave you feeling hungry and deprived, but because the DASH diet keeps you satisfied, it is much simpler to adhere to over the long term.

You will experience improved mental health.

The boost to your mood and reduced symptoms of disorders such as depression or anxiety can be attributed to the lifestyle effects of the DASH diet, such as regular exercise, moderate alcohol consumption, and cigarette avoidance. However, the nutrient-dense foods recommended by this diet are all beneficial for balancing the chemicals and hormones in your brain and body, thereby promoting mental health and well-being.

You will feel and appear youthful.

Many adherents of this diet claim that the DASH eating pattern helps them avoid some of the negative effects of aging, keeping them looking and feeling younger as the years pass. By increasing your consumption of fresh fruits and vegetables, which are rich in antioxidants, you will revitalize your skin and hair, strengthen and rejuvenate your bones, joints, and muscles, lose weight, and feel healthier.

You will live a healthier lifestyletule.

The DASH protocol isn't just about diet; it's also about taking manageable steps to control your own health and well-being. By incorporating nutrition, exercise, and healthy living into your lifestyle, you will experience a broader range of valuable benefits in addition to the health associated with DASH eating.

You will reduce your risk of developing cardiovascular disease.

Due to the DASH diet's unique ability to reduce and control blood pressure, adhering to this diet can significantly improve your body's resistance to cardiac disease. A 202 0 study indicated that the DASH diet may "substantially" reduce a person's risk for coronary heart disease, which researchers deemed to be of "great rublis health benefit" given the massive and persistent burden of coronary heart disease.

This is likely due to the fact that lower blood pressure enables your heart to function more effectively and efficiently. However, lowering blood pressure can also be beneficial for those who do not have hypertension but wish to prevent the advent of heart disease.

Researchers have discovered that the DASH diet can keep your brain alert and even prevent memory loss, thereby reducing the rate of mental decline as you age. In addition, the DASH-recommended low-fat, high-fiber diet reduces blood pressure, a known risk factor for the development of neurodegenerative diseases such as Alzheimer's and dementia.

According to research, the greatest foods for preventing mental decline include vegetables, whole grains, low-fat dairy products, legumes, and nuts – all of which make up the majority of the DASH diet.

Chapter 5: Types Of Dash Dietary Supplements

DASH, unlike other regimens, encourages a healthy, long-term lifestyle for all individuals. Exercise is essential, and there are no low-carb or fasting diet plans. In addition, the DASH diet only permits "real" or "natural" foods.

On the DASH diet menu are an abundance of nutritious fruits and vegetables, as well as low-fat and fat-free dairy products, nuts, legumes, and seeds. The adherents restrict their consumption of sodium, sugar, and foods high in saturated fat.

Try the DASH diet or diet if you want to lower your blood pressure, cholesterol, or simply shed a few excess pounds.

Followers of Dash believe that nature provides everything that humans require. It means you can consume seasonal fruits and vegetables, whole cereals, beans, lentils, and legumes, low-fat and non-fat milk, as well as natural non-dairy alternatives such as almond milk, and fresh, lean protein (fish, meat, etc.).

We also recommend measuring food with a digital scale prior to consumption. This ensures that you do not overdo.

Even "healthy" processed foods are out of place.

Physical activity is also an integral component of the DASH diet. Best results are achieved by alternating cardio with strength training (such as sprinting, running, cycling, etc.) and flexibility (such as yoga) at least three times per week.

There are two DASH diet variations:

Humans consume up to 2,6 00 milligrams (mg) of sodium per day, according to the Standard DASH Diet.

• The utmost sodium intake per day is 2 ,10 00 mg on the DASH diet.

The combination of the DASH diet and a limited sodium intake has a greater impact on blood pressure than either of these measures alone, according to experts.

As individuals reduce their salt intake, they should increase their potassium intake. Potassium relaxes blood vessels, which can reduce blood pressure. Individuals should strive to consume 8 ,700 mg of potassium daily.

The DASH diet is typically followed in two phases because it requires a change in eating patterns and the body must be retrained.

- The first phase is recommended for those who are overweight and typically lasts two weeks. During this time, a small amount of weight loss should occur.

- In the second phase, we must learn how to consume correctly by reducing our intake of saturated fats, simple sugars, and salt. In this phase, the decline in blood pressure occurs.

Which foods are best for the DASH diet?

The DASH diet instructs you to consume primarily fruits and vegetables. Five servings of vegetables and five servings of fruit per day are recommended. In addition, this plan takes carbohydrates into account and recommends seven servings of whole grains per day. Meat is consumed in moderation, with lean options and low-fat milk recommended twice daily. Two to three times a week is the recommended frequency for eating nuts and seeds.

Although the serving suggestions are quite specific, once you become accustomed to monitoring your servings for each dietary group, there is a great deal of flexibility. With a good cookbook, you will soon learn that meat and dairy products take a back seat to the many delicious and nutritious grains you can easy cook with on a daily basis.

What items are prohibited by the DASH diet?

• Beef • Bacon • Lamb

Every source of protein should be slender. When shopping, adhere to white meat, turkey meat, and fish. Low-fat yogurt and legumes are additional suitable sources of protein.

What Are Some Recipes for the DASH Diet?

The good news about the DASH diet is that many recipes can be modified to adhere to the dietary guidelines. For instance, a salad recipe could be converted into a low-fat creamy vinaigrette.

What Are Some DASH Diet Snacks?

If you are accustomed to snacking on potato crisps or candy bars, adjusting your snacking habits to DASH guidelines can be difficult at first. You will soon discover that there are numerous delicious methods to satisfy hunger pangs between meals if you exercise sufficient imagination.

Fresh vegetables and a flavorful dip are excellent methods to increase daily vegetable toppings. One of our favorite condiments is a paprika and sour cream mixture. Low-fat yogurt with fruits and granola is an excellent everyday food that can be adapted to your preferences or used to add variety to your daily diet.

What is the ideal breakfast for the DASH diet?

Instead of focusing on what is prohibited, breakfast is an excellent occasion to consume more healthy foods. For instance, one or the other may find it difficult to consume vegetables for breakfast. In this book's recipe section, you will discover the appropriate ideas.

What are the finest desserts for those following the DASH diet?

No need to be concerned if you have a sweet appetite. The DASH eating plan permits desserts. When selecting confectionery, you should pay attention to the fat content of the ingredient list. The lipids must be manufactured using whole milk and butter.

A creamy grape and marshmallow dessert prepared with just a few simple ingredients for a quick and simple dessert. Dash would also enjoy a parfait of low-fat Greek yogurt with cranberry and banana. This is discussed further in the recipe section at the conclusion of the book.

Chapter 6: How Do I Apply Dash To My Everyday Life?

This diet should be minimal in calories, sodium (salt), fat, and sugar, and it should exclude red meat.

However, the diet must include whole cereals, fruits, vegetables, and legumes.

Included in low-fat dairy products are salmon, poultry, and lean meat.

Occasionally, nuts and seeds should be incorporated. And while the optimum is to eliminate red meat, it is acceptable to consume it occasionally.

All individuals can progressively improve their eating habits by employing a series of very simple guidelines for beginning the DASH diet.

Here are some:

Double the amount of vegetables on your tray. Fresh vegetables from the market are finest.

• Put fruit in your muesli. This may include strawberries, blueberries, and avocados. In addition, you should favor grains when it comes to cereals.

• Choose a fat-free plain yogurt and add some fresh fruit to create a delectable sugar-free fruit yogurt for industrial use. They are a nutritious and intriguing option.

Smoothies are permitted on the DASH diet as long as they do not contain added sugar. If milk is used, it must be fat-free and contain citrus. Fresh or frozen vegetables that are already trimmed and ready to prepare are preferable.

Examples include broccoli, carrots, lettuce, and cauliflower. Additionally, the DASH diet emphasizes that the more vibrant the food, the better.

6 to 8 servings of grains daily.

Bread, cereal, rice, and pasta are included. It is acceptable to consume a daily portion of bread and a serving of rice or pasta. Whole grain cereals should preferably be used. This item has more fiber. Choose pasta, bread, or brown rice to fulfill your grain requirement.

Vegetables: four to five servings per day.

Vegetables are naturally abundant in fiber, nutrients, and minerals. Tomatoes, beets, and green vegetables such as broccoli are rich in minerals such as potassium and magnesium.

Consider a serving to be equivalent to a small bowl of lettuce or a half bowl of vegetables.

Four or five servings of fruit daily.

Fruits, like vegetables, are abundant in fiber, vitamins, and minerals.

Consequently, fruit is an ideal breakfast food, midday snack, or dessert.

2 to 6 servings of dairy products per day.

They are an excellent source of protein, calcium, and vitamin D.

It is crucial to choose dairy products with minimal fat content. For instance, a glass of skim milk is a lower-fat dairy product than skim milk yogurt. Because it can be complemented with fresh fruit, frozen yogurt is ideally suited for desserts.

Meat, poultry, and fish: No more than six servings per day.

Meat is an excellent source of protein, B vitamins, iron, and zinc.

Due to its high lipid content, the chicken skin should be removed.

Choose fish that is abundant in omega-6 fatty acids.

Nuts and legumes: four to five servings per week

Magnesium, potassium, protein, and fiber are abundant in almonds, sunflower or pumpkin seeds, legumes, and lentils.

Tofu can be an excellent substitute for meat, but it should be noted that soy sauce, in particular, is high in sodium and should be avoided.

Two or three servings of fats and oils per day.

You should limit your consumption of lipids and oils due to their high caloric content. These forms of fat should not exceed 6 0% of your daily caloric intake.

You must avoid consuming saturated lipids. Avoid industrial foods and baked goods at all costs.

No more than one serving of sweets per day.

This serving is already met by adding a small amount of marmalade to breakfast or a teaspoon of sugar to coffee.

Chapter 7: Understanding Calories

Calories quantify the amount of energy in sustenance. Your body needs this energy at the cellular level to complete subatomic tasks, as well as to sustain the actual tasks of daily life. A general rule of thumb: If you consume more calories than your body requires, you will likely gain weight over time. The opposite may occur if you consume less than what you truly desire. Nevertheless, there is more to it than that. Your genetics, chemistry, digestion, and activity level will also play a significant role in determining how your body weight relates to your food and calorie intake.

In the end, the majority of us consume more calories than our bodies require while also maintaining a sedentary lifestyle with negligible caloric expenditure. This mixture can result in a substantial increase in the muscle-to-fat ratio over time, particularly in the abdominal region. What impact does this have? Indeed, the Centers for Disease Control and Prevention (CDC) considers waist circumference an evaluation tool for disease risk. Men with a waist circumference greater than 8 0 inches and nonpregnant women with a waist circumference greater than 6 10 inches may be at increased risk for diabetes, hypertension, and cardiovascular disease.

Now we must consider how one pound of muscle as opposed to fat stores approximately 6 ,10 00 calories. Theoretically, if you consume 10 00 fewer calories per day than your body needs to maintain its weight, you could expect to lose approximately 2 pound of fat per week (10 00 calories multiplied by 7 days equals 6 ,10 00 calories, or 2 pound of muscle to fat ratio). This hypothesis provides a beneficial starting point for some individuals, but it also has limitations. For instance, it does not indicate that as you become more fit, your digestion will improve because a smaller body consumes fewer calories. Although this is both a misrepresentation and a conjecture, it helps explain why weight loss slows over time.

Regardless of changes to digestion that occur over time, the primary objective of any genuine weight loss effort is to create a negative energy balance, which essentially means consuming fewer calories than your body needs to maintain its current weight. A recent report from the Annals of Nutrition and Metabolism concluded that regardless of the method or strategy used to attempt weight loss, a negative energy balance remains the most important factor. The primary purpose of investigating these discoveries is to help you recognize that calories and weight loss are complicated and that we all respond to them differently.

Now that you have a better understanding of how calories function, I would like you to set them aside. Calories are an important aspect of weight management, and I'll be discussing them again, but I don't want you to become overwhelmed or obsessed with the concept.

Calories are a characteristic of sustenance. They are not what makes you feel complete, satisfied, secure, or happy. The type and amount of food you consume plays a much larger role in determining these factors. This is the type of thing I don't want you to overlook as we continue our discussion.

Then, you will learn about the appropriate portions of food and the number of servings of food you should consume to meet your daily intake goals, which will make it easier to set calorie counting for consuming the appropriate portions of a variety of foods.

Portion Control

The main component of the DASH diet is to practice healthy eating habits while supplementing with dense foods. The second most important aspect is to consume these excellent food varieties at the optimal frequency for your body's needs. After adhering to the DASH diet standards, any changes in your weight will have a substantial positive effect on your overall health and blood pressure. However, when it comes to weight loss specifically, paying a little extra attention to portion sizes will enable you to enjoy the wide variety of foods available on the DASH eating plan while still advancing toward your weight-loss objectives.

Chapter 8: So Far Conducted Research

Several studies have demonstrated that the DASH diet is advantageous for a variety of health conditions. The DASH diet has been shown to reduce blood pressure not only in those with hypertension, but also in those with normal blood pressure, even when sodium intake is not restricted. Significant reductions in blood pressure are possible if sodium intake is restricted to less than 26 00 mg per day, and even more so if sodium intake is restricted to 2 10 00 mg per day. When compared to the typical American diet, which includes a high consumption of processed and red meats, beverages with added sugar, sweets, and refined cereals, among other things, the Mediterranean diet is significantly healthier.

It has also been discovered that adhering to the DASH diet can reduce blood uric acid levels in individuals with hyperuricemia. These individuals are more likely to develop gout, a painful and inflammatory condition. The DASH diet is optimal for treating not only gout, but also high blood pressure and other cardiovascular disorders, and is therefore recommended for gout patients.

Recent meta-analyses and the Atherosclerosis Risk in Communities (ARIC) cohort, which followed over 6 ,700 individuals who developed kidney disease, indicate that adhering to the

DASH-style pattern may aid in preventing the onset of diabetes and kidney disease, respectively. Participants in the ARIC cohort who followed the DASH diet ingested an abundance of nuts, legumes, and low-fat dairy products. The consumption of red and processed meat was found to increase the risk of developing kidney disease.

Chapter 9: The Dash Diet's Characteristics

The Dash Diet is not strictly a "diet," but rather a way of eating designed to enhance one's health over a lifetime. The United States Department of Agriculture (USDA) recommends the Dietary Approach to Stop Hypertension in Its Tracks (DASH) diet as "an optimal eating plan for all Americans." According to the National Institutes of Health (NIH), the Dash diet plan does more than promote healthy eating practices. It offers suggestions for healthy alternatives to harmful foods, such as fast food and processed foods.

The following is a list of the Dash diet's characteristics:

Reduce salt consumption

Increased levels of multiple vitamins and minerals

An increase in healthy lipids

Increased fiber consumption is encouraged.

decreased intake of intoxicating beverages and coffee

Adaptable levels of sodium and caloric intake

Reduce salt consumption

The Dash diet provides guidelines for the two distinct types of food you should consume.

Sodium

The low-sodium variant of the Dash diet permits a maximum of 2 10 00 mg of sodium per day, whereas the standard Dash diet allows for a maximum of 26 00 mg of sodium per day.

Caloric

The average American diet contains up to 6 ,10 00 milligrams of sodium per day.

Increased levels of multiple vitamins and minerals

The Dash diet provides adequate quantities of all the essential vitamins and minerals that are recommended to be consumed. These include an assortment of fruits, vegetables, whole grains, and other whole foods. Magnesium and potassium are included in the diet because they both contribute to a lower or enhanced blood pressure and are rich in minerals. Inclusion in the diet also contributes to the abundance of minerals.

An increase in healthy lipids

The Dash Diet suggests restricting unhealthy lipids while increasing healthy fats. The following foods contain omega-6 fatty acids: lean meats, fish and crustaceans, low-fat dairy products, nuts and seeds. Utilizing lean meats in lieu of saturated and trans fats. Two of the ways in which consumption of healthy fats contributes to enhanced overall health are the reduction of harmful cholesterol and the elevation of beneficial cholesterol.

Increased fiber consumption is advocated

The Dash diet suggests that you can increase your daily fiber intake by consuming numerous portions of fruits, vegetables, and grains. This maintains a sensation of fullness and contributes to a reduction in blood pressure. In addition to aiding in the promotion of weight loss, a high fiber intake helps to maintain healthy blood sugar levels.

decreased intake of intoxicating beverages and coffee

On the Dash diet, it is recommended to consume less alcohol, soda, tea, and coffee due to their lack of nutritional value and propensity to contain a significant quantity of sugar. Additionally, they have been shown to increase blood pressure.

Individual sodium and calorie consumption modifications

While following the Dash diet, you have the option of consuming between 2 ,10 00 and 6 ,2 00 calories per day. Similarly, you can choose your optimal caloric intake, as well as a Dash diet with either 26 00 mg/day or 2 10 00 mg/day of sodium intake. Your weight, level of physical activity, whether you already have high blood pressure or wish to prevent it, and other factors will all depend on the caloric intake you choose.

If you are overweight already, you should choose the lower caloric consumption level on the scale. If you lead an active lifestyle, it is likely that you will choose to consume more calories. If you have high blood pressure or are at risk for developing it due to factors such as family history, you should consider adopting a lower-sodium diet. You may wish to consult your primary care physician in order to ascertain the optimal sodium-to-calorie ratio for your needs.

Chapter 10: Common Dietary Contributors To Hypertension

The absence of hypertension in your family history and other hypertensive risk factors does not rule out the possibility that other factors are causing your health problems. Typically, this determinant is the food we eat. There are numerous foods that can cause your blood pressure to skyrocket, and consuming them frequently makes it difficult to control this condition. Among the meals you must avoid are the following:

Fast cuisine is the primary cause of your elevated blood pressure. If you frequently visit the drive-through window, you are undoubtedly consuming more sodium than your body requires. Learning how to limit eating out to special occasions or finding other meals (such as freezer meals) that can be prepared swiftly and are nutritious will make a significant difference.

Deli meats: Processed picnic meats and deli meats can be extremely high in sodium. With salt, these kinds of meats can be preserved, seasoned, and even cured. In fact, a 2 ounce serving of certain lunch meats may contain as much as 10 00 milligrams of sodium. And if you add cucumbers, condiments, cheese, and bread, you really pile on the salt.

If you are really watching your sodium intake, you should be cautious about all varieties of pizza, including frozen pizza. Crust, tomato sauce, cured meats, and cheese can add up to a significant amount of sodium. But even worse are refrigerated pizzas. In order to preserve its flavor, the manufacturer frequently adds a substantial amount of salt. A frozen meat and cheese or cheese pizza may contain over 700 milligrams of sodium per serving.

Salt is required to preserve any form of food, including pickles. This prevents the food from decaying and can make it edible for a much extended period of time. However, this means that even healthful foods, such as cucumber, can absorb sodium when transformed into pickles. The longer the vegetables remain in the canning liquids, the greater their sodium content will be. In fact, a whole spear of dill pickles can contain up to 6 90 milligrams of sodium.

Canned soup: Despite the fact that canned soups are quick and straightforward to prepare on days when you are pressed for time, they are loaded with sodium. Some soups contain as much as 900 milligrams of sodium per half-cup serving. This implies that you could consume more than 2 grams of sodium per can.

Products canned and bottled with tomatoes: Tomato products with added sodium are extremely problematic for those with hypertension. A half-cup serving of marinara sauce may contain 8 00 milligrams of sodium, whereas a cup of tomato juice typically contains over 600 milligrams. If you include these in your diet, search for versions with low or reduced sodium content.

Sugar: Consuming too much sugar is associated with increased weight gain and obesity, as well as elevated blood pressure. Regardless of age, sugar found in numerous products, but particularly in sugar-sweetened beverages, can contribute to obesity in humans. Moreover, those who are obese and overweight will be more likely to have hypertension. The U.S. Department of Agriculture does not set a daily sugar intake limit, but the American Heart Association recommends that women consume no more than 6 teaspoons and men consume no more than 9 teaspoons.

Those with elevated blood pressure should reduce their consumption of saturated fats and avoid trans fats found in chicken skin and packaged foods. This includes butter, red meat, full-fat dairy products, and poultry skin. Small quantities of trans fats can be found in dairy products and fatty meats. However, these trans fats are most prevalent in packaged and prepared foods, which should be avoided.

Alcohol: Drinking one or two glasses on occasion can help lower blood pressure, but excessive drinking will have the opposite effect and raise blood pressure. In addition, long-term excessive drinking increases the risk of cancer, even if it is done occasionally. According to information released by the Mayo Clinic, individuals who consume more than three alcoholic beverages in a single sitting may experience sudden increases in blood pressure. This event may be temporary until it turns into a habit.

Chapter 11: The Influence And Strength Of Dash Diet

Whether you are a child, a student, a professional, a caregiver, or a retiree, the challenges of modern life have compelled you to lead a balanced existence. The modern era is swift, and we have no time to delve into the specifics of techniques that help us live a healthy existence. Now, with the advancement of technology, it is much simpler to conduct research on a variety of health-related topics, but has this eliminated the need for expert analysis by a medical representative? Well, I'd say NO!

Internet can be very confusing, and you may become disoriented in the global web of health information. In Chapter II, we will begin by analyzing the Dash Diet's Nutrition Chart. In addition, we will discuss three essential aspects of the Dash Diet.

Positive Effects of the Dash Diet

The Difficulties of the Dash Diet

The Comprehensive View of Dash Diet

Dash Diet – Nutrition Chart EXPLAINED

Let's start with the Nutrition Chart, shall we?

As you can see, the Dash Diet incorporates a wide variety of foods that provide essential macronutrients – carbohydrates, proteins, and fats.

Depending on your health conditions, gender, and age, the Dash Diet reduces your sodium intake from food.

Its formulation includes proportions of a variety of colorful foods, including spinach, broccoli, lentils, salmon, chicken breast, tuna, yogurt, almonds, raisins, pistachios, avocados, dark chocolate, mangoes, oranges, and more.

These nutrients are the primary sources of calcium, potassium, and magnesium, which help prevent and manage hypertension, cholesterol, diabetes, and weight.

Health Tip: SALT is the primary source of sodium in our diet and is one of the ingredients that can cause elevated blood pressure. Adding a pinch of SALT (but no more) can help soothe your taste receptors and get you through the first few days of reducing your sodium intake.

The two most important aspects of the Dash diet to consider for measurable results are:

Depending on your medical condition, you must either limit or eliminate your alcohol consumption.

Sweets and flavored foods must be avoided for optimal results.

I. Positive Effects of the Dash Diet

Dash Diet is well-known as a family-friendly diet. This nutrition plan can be followed by individuals of all ages, including children, adults, and senior citizens, and it promotes the health of the entire family.

2 .) A Wholesome Diet – Dash Diet

The Dash Diet encourages the consumption of all three macronutrients: carbohydrates, proteins, and lipids. The purpose of this diet is to provide for your primary meals – breakfast, lunch, and dinner – as well as your snacking requirements throughout the day. In such a diet, you tend to consume a variety of healthy foods, which reduces your likelihood of consuming garbage or unhealthy foods.

2.) Maintain Blood Pressure Management

With today's stressful lifestyle, it can be extremely difficult to adhere to a dietary plan, let alone a nutrition plan. The consumption of whole grains, fruits, and vegetables reduces hunger, particularly when consumed in modest amounts throughout the day. Potassium, calcium, and magnesium-rich diets are essential for maintaining normal blood pressure levels.

The amount of sodium required by the human body is currently a source of confusion for the majority of individuals. So, you may ask me, AuthorName> is sodium not as essential as other nutritional components?

Certainly, it is! Sodium is an essential element for the human body, and its consumption is more of a concern than a query. Dash Diet is formulated to provide the optimal quantity of sodium, which facilitates vital bodily functions and prevents the accumulation of additional fluids. High levels of sodium can lead to fluid retention, which in turn raises blood pressure.

The NIH has discovered that the Dash Diet can reduce a person's blood pressure in JUST 2 8 days – Incredible Fact

6 .) The NEW Extra Advantage of the Dash Diet - Cholesterol Management

Dash Diet is widely recognized as the MOST EXAMINED topic of its kind. Researchers discovered that this varied diet not only aids in lowering blood pressure but also aids in lipid management. How, you may ask? Fibers perform an important role in controlling cholesterol levels. The Dash nutrition plan calls for the consumption of high-fibre foods such as brown rice, oats, barley, millet, and other whole-wheat products.

A recent variation in the Dash study revealed that the consumption of high-fat dairy products in the diet could actually reduce the levels of bad cholesterol in affected individuals. Hey! Before you call me crazy for contradicting myself, let me tell you that, in addition to the new findings, it was also observed that two individuals who followed the Dash diet with two distinct patterns of consuming high-fat and low-fat dairy products had the same blood pressure-lowering effects. This is what I call DASH sorcery!

Men should consume between 6 0 and 6 8 grams of fiber per day, while women should consume between 20 and 210 grams per day.

8 .) The Weight Control Program

Over the years, the Dash Diet has emerged as a weight reduction program and is said to have a significant impact on individuals battling weight issues such as obesity. In addition to its primary purpose of reducing cardiac problems by lowering blood pressure, the Dash Diet has measurable effects on weight. Consuming fruits and vegetables at regular intervals keeps you satisfied, which helps you control your calorie consumption. However, if you're seeking a rapid weight loss solution, I wouldn't recommend the Dash Diet.

According to the World Health Organization (WHO), the combination prevents dangerous diseases like cancer.

Diet and exercise can do marvels for your body. If you engage in any form of exercise — cardio, gym, aerobics, Zumba, etc. — and are uncertain about which diet to choose, choose the DASH DIET, which is the best.

Important Note: I would like to draw your attention to the fact that no matter what fast weight loss plan you follow or how much you starve yourself to lose those extra pounds, there will be negative consequences. A major advantage of following the Dash Diet is that despite the modest weight loss results, it will have a long-lasting, nourishing influence.

II. The Dash Diet's Complexities Complexities? Did you just repeat complexities Cage? Yes, I did! Unfortunately, every diet has disadvantages, and the Dash Diet is no exception. While the regimen has been endorsed by the world's leading health organizations, I would like to draw your attention to two significant complications.

2 .) Taste Issues – Burg! Where has the SALT gone?

Families and individuals who have always preferred less SALT in their food will not experience any difficulty, but those who are accustomed to adding SALT to their prepared meals may experience a moment of irritability. You may initially find it difficult to tolerate the flavor, but you will eventually get used to it. I assure you that a little perseverance will yield enormous benefits.

2.) Calorie Check – The Highs and Lows Are Horrifying! This one is undoubtedly terrifying, and I have experienced it. The older version of myself carried a schedule and a meter to ensure that I did not consume more than what was intended. Oh well, that's the past! However, you are aware that the formulation of the DASH Diet is quite precise, and that all you need is a nutrition plan tailored to your lifestyle. I would advise against going overboard with the calorie check thingy, as doing so could hinder your health objectives, resulting in NO results at all.

III. The Greater Context of the DASH Diet

I believe that behind every action, minor or large, there is always a larger picture, and committing to the Dash Diet is no exception. No matter what your objective is or how hard you've worked to achieve it, you must remember one thing: Your health is not just for you, but for your loved ones as well...

It is said that the Dash Diet is one of the most successful diets, with novel benefits added to its original design. It is widely recognized and utilized due to its enduring benefits such as longevity, its affordability (certainly does not burn a hole in your wallet), and its all-encompassing approach to leading an active lifestyle.

Are you prepared to produce and enjoy some delicious and nourishing foods? Then, let's proceed to the following sections where I will introduce you to some nutritious recipes.

Chapter 12: Workouts For The Growth Of The Biceps

The BICEPS CURL BAR

This exercise is excellent for strengthening the entire arm and biceps. To perform this exercise, a bar must be loaded with an average amount of weight. Holding the boom in its original position, lift the weight to your chest and then carefully lower it to your thighs. Continue the sequence until you are done.

ALTERNATING DUMBBELL CURL

This exercise is designed to strengthen the triceps. It is optimal for any exercise designed to build muscle mass. To perform the exercise, you will need to grasp two moderately-weighted dumbbells. One hand retains the massive object while the other hand executes the entire trajectory. After the weight has been lowered under controlled conditions, the arm returns to its original position and the other arm lifts. The cycle is repeated until the end of the exercise.

PRECEPTOR CURL

This exercise is excellent for enhancing the size, definition, and strength of the outer biceps.

This task can only be performed by a well-known bank. It is named after Mr. Olympia Larry Scott, who popularized it. To accomplish this, a bar must be loaded with weight. Weight must be enclosed in parentheses. Once the arms are supported by the supports, grasp the bar at the same distance as the shoulders.

Next, raise the weight until your head touches it. Carry on with the series.

CONCENTRATION CURL

This is an isolated exercise that provides your biceps definition. It requires a challenging effort and eight to ten repetitions. The limb holding the formidable is supported by a flat bank. Lifting the weight for two seconds controls the flexion movement. After that, the weight is lowered gradually.

Chapter 13: Exercising For The Growth Of The Triceps

Tricep Extension While Bar-Sitting

A robust arm is possible if the triceps are well-developed. Open a grasp bar and lower your weight to accomplish this. Increase the weight until you reach the beginning position once the bar reaches your back.

Pulling Triceps Using a Pulley

The milestone with pulley is an excellent exercise for triceps development. It helps build muscle mass and gives the arm definition. You must locate a weight that you can lift comfortably. Once you are capable of doing so, place your hands on the pulleys and carefully lower the weight. Keep your forearms straight in order to prevent injury-causing, jerky movements.

Triceps Punch

This exercise is beneficial for the triceps because it is a "horseshoe" exercise. The hand that is gripping the formidable is also holding the elbow along the trunk. As soon as the arm is in place, the hand holding the formidable moves rearward. The hand holding the formidable then extends the arm a second time before returning it to its initial position. Repeat the steps until both hands have been completed.

One-Hand Triceps Extension

This exercise is fantastic for developing the outer triceps. The method is straightforward. A formidable individual must have a light-to-moderate build and carry his head aloft. Once the weight is behind the head, the arm must be extended and the weight must be lowered under control.

Description of the Dash Diet

In the United States, the incidence of Morbid Hypertension increased at an alarming rate in 2 992. In order to combat this issue, the DASH Diet was developed. Now, after years of extensive research conducted by numerous health institutions, the DASH Diet is being actively promoted by various branches of the United States government. Not only is it recommended for people with morbid hypertension, but it is also viewed as a model for all Americans to follow in order to prevent a variety of conditions whose causes are primarily attributable to dietary and lifestyle choices.

The DASH (Dietary Approaches to Stop Hypertension) Diet suggests the following dietary modifications:

The consumption of more fruits, vegetables, whole cereals, and low-fat dairy products rises.

Reduce the consumption of red meat and replace it with alternative sources of protein such as seafood, poultry, nuts, and beans.

Not exceeding 6 ,200 mg of salt per day.

Three tablespoons of sugar per day maximum.

A daily limit of two alcoholic beverages.

No more than three caffeinated beverages per day (this includes soft drinks like cola and some energy drinks).

Two groups of individuals who were encouraged to follow the DASH Diet have been studied. The first group served as a control and consisted of individuals with no underlying or pre-existing medical conditions. The second group consisted of individuals who had already been diagnosed with hypertension. Both categories included men and women between the ages of 8 8 and 86 .

In both instances, the results indicated a significant reduction in blood pressure over the duration of the study. In the control group, systolic blood pressure decreased by 6mm Hg, while diastolic blood pressure decreased by 6 mm Hg. In the hypertensive group, the reduction in systolic blood pressure was 2 2 mm Hg, while the reduction in diastolic blood pressure was 6 mm Hg.

Both of these outcomes are impressive. Such a significant reduction in blood pressure would be of immense benefit to the individuals by lowering their risk for a variety of conditions, including heart failure, kidney disease, coronary heart disease, and atherosclerosis.

It is essential to be aware that even the healthiest foods may contain concealed sources of sugars, salt, and fats. Always examine the packaging for sodium preservatives, corn syrups, and saturated fats, and whenever possible, fresh produce is preferable to packaged foods.

The DASH Diet is not a fad that promises rapid weight loss; rather, it is a philosophy of healthy eating combined with lifestyle adjustments that is meant to be sustainable, enjoyable, and will ultimately result in enormous health benefits.

How Can Smoothies Be Used for the Dash Diet?

After selecting and purchasing a blender, the next query is what to put inside. This boils down to individual preferences and preferences. However, there are a few things to keep in mind when making your own smoothies.

Consider balancing sweet and sour fruits to achieve the desired flavor when producing the flavor. Adding frozen fruit or fibrous fruits such as bananas or pineapples to your mélange will result in a creamier texture in the final product. Consider adding water-rich fruits and vegetables such as cantaloupe, oranges, apples, and carrots, rather than simply adding more ice, if you desire a watery consistency.

It is ideal to purchase organic fruits and vegetables, as they do not contain any of the harmful chemicals associated with modern pesticides.

In order to create novel and interesting flavor combinations that are also healthier, you may wish to include ingredients other than fruits and vegetables. For instance, flax seeds will increase the fiber content of your smoothie without altering its flavor, and kefir can be used as a yogurt substitute because it contains more beneficial microorganisms and nutrients. If you want to increase the protein content, you can add nuts or protein powder. However, protein powder should always be added at the conclusion of the blending process because it causes the smoothie to become foamy. Is your smoothie excessively sour? Then, honey is added.

The combinations are limitless, and if you are unsure of what you want, a quick Internet search will yield a multitude of free recipes that you can attempt at your leisure.

Smoothies are without a doubt the quickest and simplest way to alter your eating habits for the better. They are delicious, nutritious, and incredibly simple to prepare. The ingredients are easily accessible and inexpensive. With all of these benefits, there is no reason why smoothies shouldn't be an integral part of everyone's diet.

Chapter 14: Dash Diet To Shrink The Waistline

The DASH diet consists of two phases. The regimen begins with a 2 8 -day Phase 2 that assists with blood sugar regulation. In this phase, satisfying appetite and managing cravings are also important objectives.

Phase 2 entails making the DASH diet a way of life. The DASH diet is not a one-time solution for achieving health and fitness objectives. Yes, achieving slimmer waistlines in a brief period of time is effective. However, the greatest results for your waistline and overall health are obtained when the DASH diet becomes a way of life. Consequently, Phase 2 alters how you view and approach food and consuming in general.

DASH for weight reduction Phase 2

This is the first two weeks of the regimen that will help you lose a significant amount of belly fat. During this time, you will also be lighter and experience lighterness.

The most essential aspect of this phase is avoiding starchy foods high in sugar. This dietary modification will primarily regulate your blood sugar level. This alone will generate numerous benefits, including:

Enhanced insulin regulation

Effectively suppresses appetite

Have more vitality

Regulate hunger effectively

Feel satiated longer

Heighten adipose metabolism

Improve cardiovascular health Improve blood flow

Enhance cognitive abilities (thinking, deciding, etc.).

Better emotional management

The enumeration continues.

Currently, you should focus on consuming more verdant greens and cruciferous vegetables. Due to the high levels of natural sugars, you should also avoid eating whole cereals and fruits at this time.

The primary focus of Phase 2 would be fresh salads with low-sodium, low-fat dressings. When it comes to salad dressings, yogurt will be your best companion.

Meats and other healthful protein sources are permitted during Phase 2 . If you weary of green salads, you can opt for sandwiches without bread. Consider a lean burger with a low-fat dressing, an abundance of vegetables such as tomatoes and cabbage, no ketchup, buns, or cheddar.

This phase also affords you the chance to sample seafood such as wild salmon and tuna. poultry is also delicious.

Losing a few centimeters does not require a monotonous diet of salads. You can still enjoy dining. You must simply give up pasta, bread, toast, pastries, and other starchy foods. No cake either. But what's a slice of cake compared to looking nice in clothes that are two to three sizes smaller than what you're wearing today?

The fundamentals of Phase 2 are:

No carbohydrate

Nothing made with cornmeal

No vegetables either

Neither whole cereals nor

Up to 6 ounces of protein per day, but only from lean sources.

Consume four to five servings of lentils or legumes each week.

Additionally, healthy lipids should be included. This includes plant-based lipids such as seeds and nuts. Fruits abundant in healthful monounsaturated fats are also excellent options. Avocados are also abundant in beta-carotene, lutein, and vitamin E. These are potent antioxidants that can improve your health even further. These can also help you eliminate those annoying belly fats more quickly.

Olive oil, nut oils, and canola oil are additional plant-based sources of healthy lipids. These will be staples in your salad dressing recipes, particularly during Phase 2 . These oils are also ideal for sautéing or frying (yes, frying) lean proteins such as pan-seared salmon or chicken breasts.

Additionally, fatty fish such as mackerel and salmon are excellent sources.

Phase 2 of DASH for weight loss

Following Phase 2 's 2 8 -day duration, the same food inventory will be used for the subsequent phase. Additional nutritious foods will be reintroduced into your diet. This means that you will now be able to consume nutritious starches. A few fruits and sweet delights are now permitted.

Your new diet will consist of six to eight daily servings of whole grains. Best options include breads and pasta made with whole grains. Cereals made with whole grains are also among your options.

As mentioned, fruits are now permitted. They are available fresh or frozen. Four to five portions of fruit should be consumed daily. Fruits with low sugar content and high nutrient content are excellent options. Examples are berries and avocados.

Limit dairy consumption to yogurt and low-fat milk. daily servings are between 2 and 6 , the same as in Phase 2 .

Sugars are now permitted, but should be restricted. Avoid unhealthy desserts, such as those containing white or refined sugar. You are only allowed 6 to 8 servings per week. That translates to a tiny serving of frozen yogurt instead of traditional ice cream, a couple of bites of cake or pie, or a couple of tablespoons of custard. You can savor some of the old candies in smaller quantities. It is preferable to also make healthful substitutions. For example, choose a cake made with dark chocolate (at least 710 % cacao) rather than a traditional chocolate cake. Instead of conventional snack products, select granola. Instead of conventional chocolate confectionary, choose a bar of dark chocolate.

Alcohol is permissible in the diet, but those who do not consume it regularly are better off without it. One glass of wine is equivalent to one serving of produce. You may substitute your daily fruit serving for the small quantity of wine.

As you now know, the DASH diet provides a basic diet and lifestyle to adhere to in order to lower blood pressure. Nonetheless, there is a reason why this regimen is ranked number one. In fact, the DASH diet can bring a variety of health benefits into your existence. It is remarkable what fruits, vegetables, whole grains, and healthful fats can accomplish. Below, we will examine the numerous advantages of the DASH diet in greater detail.

Reduce Your Blood Force

Obviously, this benefit is self-evident. The DASH diet was designed specifically to reduce blood pressure. When you begin to monitor your sodium intake, you will notice a decrease in your blood pressure. In addition, the diet helps individuals maintain a healthy balance of cholesterol and triglycerides that can be harmful to the body. In exchange, this aids in the prevention of atherosclerosis. Simply put, this is when your arteries constrict and cause an increase in blood pressure. This can be detrimental because it strains the cardiovascular system.

Weight Loss

Initially, the DASH diet was not designed to promote weight loss. As scientists studied the DASH diet, they discovered that it had a terrific side effect for those attempting to lose weight. People began losing weight primarily due to the elimination of what are known as empty carbohydrates. In case you were oblivious, the empty carbohydrates we consume are also devoid of calories. Not only are you consuming excess calories, but these carbohydrates also raise your blood glucose levels and cause instability. When the equilibrium is lost, diabetes is often the result. Obesity rates begin to decline once people begin focusing on their caloric intake and ingesting fruits and vegetables in a healthier manner.

Health of the Heart and Cholesterol

The main focus of the DASH diet is on lowering blood pressure, but the reason why this is so essential is because high blood pressure poses a significant threat to the heart. When you place excessive tension and strain on your arteries and blood vessels, you increase your risk of suffering from a heart attack or stroke. On the DASH diet, fiber consumption is increased. As you consume more fiber, your body's cholesterol levels begin to equalize. Consequently, the plaque that can accumulate around the heart begins to diminish. The more healthy you are, the less likely you are to develop complications from heart disease and other diseases that affect your vital organs.

Kidney Benefits

In addition to the benefits listed above, studies have shown a positive correlation between the DASH diet and the prevention of kidney stones. Due to the composition of the DASH diet, excess mineral deposits that can contribute to kidney stones are prevented. In case you were unaware, kidney stones are notoriously excruciating. In addition to the agony, the organ's normal functions are also compromised. Frequently, kidney stones are associated with a high daily sodium intake. This can cause kidney failure owing to dehydration on its own. When organs are deprived of adequate hydration, they begin to overwork and eventually fail. If you already have chronic kidney disease, the DASH diet may not be the optimal choice for you. Instead of adopting the DASH diet, you should consult your physician immediately to determine the optimal diet for your condition.

Osteoporosis Avoidance

On the DASH diet, your nutrient intake will likely increase due to the foods you consume. This results in increased levels of protein, potassium, and even calcium. All of these are known to help prevent or delay the onset of osteoporosis. By consuming the necessary nutrients, the body can build robust bones. The DASH diet includes foods such as whole cereals, leafy greens, fruits, and milk as a source of protein. All of these help individuals construct a solid foundation, in addition to receiving the other incredible benefits of the DASH diet.

Caring for Diabetes

One of the main benefits of the DASH diet is eliminating unnecessary starchy foods and empty carbohydrates. They contain inert calories that provide minimal to no essential nutrients for daily activities. When you avoid simple carbohydrates, you reduce the amount of sugar in your bloodstream. The unfortunate aspect of simple carbohydrates is their rapid absorption by the body. In turn, this severely disrupts the insulin and glucose levels in our bodies. Unfortunately, when this occurs, it leads to diabetes. Diabetes can also result in cardiovascular disease and obesity. Fortunately, you can take the initial measures to prevent it from occurring in the first place by beginning your DASH diet.

Cancer Treatment

In some instances, scientists discovered that the DASH diet has a definite impact on certain types of cancer. As you will discover in later chapters, the DASH diet consists of a variety of fruits and vegetables. These foods contain more vitamins, antioxidants, and fiber than others. It has been discovered that these substances can neutralize the effects of free radicals. Free radicals are cellular respiration's byproducts. This is caused by the mutation of healthy cells and results in the spread of certain malignancies. By consuming these nutrients, you reduce the likelihood of this happening in your body.

Reduced Appetite

One of the non-health benefits of the DASH diet is that the foods tend to keep individuals fuller for longer. This is extremely beneficial, particularly if you are using this regimen to lose weight. On a diet, you will consume fruits and vegetables rich in fiber in addition to lean proteins. According to studies, these nutrients keep you fuller for longer. In turn, this will result in reduced daily caloric intake. This may not be a health benefit, but it is still beneficial if you intend to follow this regimen for life. Who, after all, desires to constantly feel hungry?

Increased Vitality

Consider the regimen you are currently following. Do you ever experience daytime lethargy? This may be the result of consuming too many toxic foods. You will learn how to balance your diet and, as a result, provide your body with the nutrients it requires to increase your energy levels while following the DASH diet. You may find that you have more vitality throughout the day if you consume whole grains, lean meats, and fruits and vegetables. In addition to diet, exercise is also recommended.

According to studies, an increase in regular exercise enhances endurance and provides an energy boost. As you begin to balance your energy, you will also be able to balance your sleep, which is the key to enhancing your energy levels significantly.

Mood Improvements

Everyone has terrible days. This is a consequence of being human. However, research indicates that when people change their diet and begin exercising, they feel better about their physical appearance. When you have a positive self-perception, your self-esteem and confidence soar. In addition, the benefits include enhanced cognitive function and reduced tension. It is incredible how life-changing healthy behaviors can be. When you begin to feel better about yourself on the outside and the inside, this could contribute to an improvement in cognitive function and an expansion of your social circle. When you alter your lifestyle, you may wish to inform your acquaintances and loved ones. Regardless of the lifestyle or health decisions you make in your lifetime, a strong support system is essential.

Clearly, the DASH diet has numerous extraordinary benefits. We hope at least one of these examples resonated with you. Obviously, not every diet is suitable for everyone. In the following chapter, we will examine the benefits and drawbacks of the DASH diet. In this chapter, we hope to persuade you to adopt the DASH diet immediately in order to better your life.

Chapter 15: The Dash Diet For Lowering Blood Pressure, Losing Weight, And Achieving Optimal Health

You are already aware that the DASH diet was designed to reduce elevated blood pressure, which, if uncontrolled, leads to stroke or heart disease. Let's examine how the DASH diet assists in the management of hypertension, diabetes, weight loss, and metabolic syndrome.

The DASH Diet and Hypertension

It has been demonstrated that strict adherence to the DASH diet while limiting sodium intake to the minimal recommendation of 2 ,10 00 mg has a direct effect on high blood pressure. According to extensive studies conducted by the NIH, combining certain nutrients with a minimal sodium intake has yielded substantial benefits. The Mayo Clinic accentuates this further by stating that if you follow the DASH diet for two weeks, your blood pressure can drop by several points. Over time, your blood pressure is likely to decrease by 8 to 2 8 points, effectively reducing your health risks.

It is recommended that you follow the DASH diet if you are at risk of developing high blood pressure due to underlying risk factors such as ethnicity (African-Americans are at high risk), lifestyle choices (such as a high sodium intake or smoking), or weight (obesity is a major risk factor for hypertension).

DASH Diet and Weight Loss

DASH advocates consuming significantly less fat than the typical American diet. This indicates that it contains fewer calories. This diet eliminates and limits unhealthy lipids, fast food, fried foods, and highly processed foods. It emphasizes healthy lipids such as saturated fats and healthy saturated fats such as omega 6 fats, which are beneficial to the body and aid in weight loss. These are typically found in low-calorie foods. The high fiber content of the majority of foods recommended by the DASH diet is another important factor in weight loss because fibers promote satiety and assist digestion, allowing the body to eliminate wastes while slowing the absorption of sugar and fat. This facilitates efficient insulin regulation and response, thereby reducing the risk and symptoms of metabolic syndrome.

High consumption of raw vegetables and fruits results in high vitamin C and antioxidant levels. Vitamin C is essential for reducing the effects of stress, as it decreases the amount of cortisol produced. Additionally, this hormone is accountable for fat storage in the abdominal region. Therefore, what you consume will not be stored as abdominal fat. In addition, vitamin C is a building block of L-carnitine, which is essential for lipid transport. When the body receives a signal that it no longer requires fat, it converts it into glucose for energy. Vitamin C is required for the body to produce L-carnitine naturally. This means that vitamin C must be consumed daily for it to contribute to weight loss, as its primary function is battling infection and repairing damaged cells.

The DASH diet also recommends individualized caloric intake based on a person's weight loss objectives, current weight, body shape, and level of physical activity. This diet prevents you from consuming so few calories that you run the risk of losing lean muscle tissue rather than fat, while ensuring you get enough nutrients to support your activity level.

DASH diet and Heart Disease

When you have excessive blood pressure, metabolic syndrome, and type 2 diabetes, it is likely that you will develop heart disease. Due to the fact that the DASH diet addresses all of these conditions, it can also reduce your risk of heart disease. Even if you do not currently suffer from any of these conditions, this diet is an excellent choice. Heart disease is the leading cause of mortality in the United States. A diet limited in unhealthy fats and high in healthy fats and fiber is recommended by health professionals to improve heart health. DASH is recommended by the American Heart Association as a heart-healthy diet. In addition to boosting heart health, this diet also reduces the risk of kidney stones and improves colon and digestive health.

The DASH Diet and the Development of Metabolic Syndrome

A group of symptoms associated with insulin and adiposity is referred to as the metabolic syndrome. This syndrome is referred to as pre-diabetes because, if left untreated, it leads to type 2 diabetes. High blood sugar, a large waist circumference, elevated HDL, and elevated triglycerides are common indicators of metabolic syndrome. The DASH diet can eliminate these undesirable side effects. The DASH diet includes a reduction in unhealthy lipids and an increase in healthy fats and fiber, which are beneficial for lowering triglyceride and HDL cholesterol levels. The nutrients you obtain from the DASH diet, coupled with the abdominal fat loss you experience, significantly reduce metabolic syndrome, allowing you to enjoy optimal health.

DASH Diet and Type 2 Diabetes

U.S. News and World Report ranked the DASH diet as the greatest diet for combating Type 2 diabetes and for those at risk of developing diabetes. It has been demonstrated that this diet can substantially reduce both the symptoms and severity of diabetes. In some instances, the dietary modification associated with this diet has been effective in reversing the condition. The reason for this is straightforward. The DASH diet consists of nutrients that improve the health of diabetics. Nuts, for instance, help diabetics control their glucose levels, while a high fiber content will delay the absorption of sugar, thereby preventing blood sugar fluctuations. All of the vegetables and fruits in the DASH diet are rich in antioxidants that aid in the prevention and reduction of Type 2 diabetes complications. The DASH diet can also aid in the prevention of type 2 diabetes by promoting weight loss, particularly abdominal obesity, which is responsible for insulin resistance.

Chapter 16: The Mystery Behind Dash Diet Food

Be waru of fad diet trends. There are valid reasons to exclude certain foods from your diet, but in many cases, people resort to novelty diets to lose weight rather than because of a specific medical condition. The greatest disadvantage of fad diets is that they do not alter long-term food habits and are unsustainable.

The DASH Diet is your ticket to better health if you're looking for an evidence-based, easy-to-follow diet that you can maintain indefinitely. The secret? It is proven. Due to its name, Dietary Approach to Stop Hypertension, the research for this diet began as an effort to reduce blood pressure. But what's really interesting is that after multiple research trials, it was found to promote weight loss, diabetic control, and bone health.

Eating the DASH diet is also sustainable (i.e., you can maintain it long-term), something that many fad diets cannot claim. We all desire instant gratification from time to time, but eating well is a lifetime commitment. Focus on adding healthy foods to your diet, such as a variety of fresh fruits and vegetables, fat-free or low-fat milk products, whole grains, and lean meats, rather than relying on supplements.

Simple Tir for Beginning DASH Todau:

Include fruit, protein, and fiber in your morning meal. Add blueberries or banana slices to your oatmeal. Tor topped with a handful of chopped almonds.

At lunchtime, add protein to a salad – try 6 -8 ounces of seared salmon or chicken on a bed of mixed green with a vinaigrette dre. Or tor salad with dried cranberries, one tableroon of sunflower seeds, and cottage cheese.

Prerare extra vegetables ahead. Steam, grill, or sauté a larger quantity of your preferred vegetable (rinash, zushini, broccoli, rerrer, onion, or green bean). Use within the next two to three days for lunch or dinner, or to incorporate into a grain dish.

Examine the food on your tray. Balance your diet by consuming half fruits and vegetables, a small amount of protein, and a small amount of high-fiber grains.

Exercise in conjunction with a healthy diet is a great way to lose weight. The ineffective method of starving yourself to death and doing nothing is not an effective way to lose those unwanted love handles. You can even get sisk if uou do not do it rrorerlu.

Whether we like it or not, we must consume food. Like sar rart, our major organs may not function effectively without fuel (food). If we stop eating properly, we begin to lose oxygen in our bloodstreams, which can cause various health issues. To remain healthy, we must consume the nutrient-dense foods our bodies require.

Numerous individuals have discovered the advantages of drinking vegetable juice. It has been suggested that certain vegetables can help combat illness and even cancer. These characters are not only becoming healthier, but have also begun to lose weight.

Vegetable juice is great due to its salorie sontent. A glass of vegetable juice contains only 8 6 calories. It is rich in vitamins and nutrients that can help you live longer and healthier. However, it is recommended that you make your own vegetable juice at home. Processed commercial vegetable juice contains a high sodium concentration. To avoid this, you can simply purchase an electric juicer and enjoy your juice in the convenience of your own home.

Another benefit of vegetable juice is that you do not need to peel, dice, or easy cook the vegetables before you can enjoy your meal. Using a juicer, you can juice a whole carrot or even add some kale, and then consume the liquid. You san even add some srises like sauenne pepper, cardamom, or allsrise. The addition of a dash of rise to your vegetable juice can boost your metabolism and help you lose weight quickly.

Some reorle attempt juising for five full days per month. This may help them lose weight by promoting detoxification. This eliminates and melts away those undesirable lipids. Before beginning a diet, however, it is prudent to consult a physician for precautionary purposes.

Disrupt Your Dieting Routine

Instead of focusing on the latest fad diet, you should focus on consuming foods that will help you lose weight and maintain a healthy weight, as well as aid in the fight against chronic diseases such as diabetes, heart disease, and even cancer.

You can incorporate as many nutritious foods as you can imagine into a diet rich in flavor, satisfaction, and vitality without ever having to consider your waistline again. Until they give it a try, this statement appears to be a novelty to a large number of individuals.

Certainly, this means spitting out fast food and soda. In the long term, however, you won't be interested in these foods at all! However, there are numerous foods that can easily substitute for fast food and sugary beverages. For example, you can eat homemade shiitake mushroom nasho or pizza for dinner at any time without gaining weight, as long as you prepare it yourself and use the proper ingredients.

What are The Correct Components?

The proper ingredients to use when preparing food for weight loss and healthy living do not arrive in a bag or a box. Make your own chili from scratch using a combination of pinto and black beans along with tomatoes, chile flakes, bell peppers, sugar, chili powder, and a pinch of salt.

Instead of frying frozen or previously cooked French fries, cut your own potatoes into wedges, sprinkle them with olive oil and a pinch of salt, and roast them in the oven. Another simple way to replace a less-than-healthy product is to replace white rice with whole wheat varieties and use brown or wild rice.

Here are some things you can do to relieve yourself of a negative mindset:

Change your negative habit to a good one:

I am aware this is challenging, but not impossible. Do you always consume more food than you should? The majority of people overeat not because they are hungry, but because they derive emotional solace from food. Since no other food would provide more enjoyment and comfort than junk food, these individuals consume as much of it as possible. You cannot expect to lose weight until you break this unhealthy dietary pattern.

The first step in kicking this habit is realizing that food cannot comfort you in any way; if you're depressed, frustrated, or simply bored, you need to find other methods to turn your life's negativity into positivity. If you are bored on Sunday because you have nothing to do, why not go swimming, play basketball, or engage in any other activity you enjoy?

If you keep yourself occupied with numerous activities, you won't even realize how and when time has passed! In addition, you won't feel the need to consume unhealthy food! Plu, if you remain active, you will also be able to lose weight and become physically fit. What a way to slay two birds with one stone!

Think like a champion:

Stop constantly thinking like a loser and start thinking like a winner! Believe it or not, if you change your mindset and attitude, you can accomplish anything! One thing you can do is to create two lists: one detailing your various assets and abilities, and the other outlining the obstacles and roadblocks preventing you from reaching your weight loss goal.

Chapter 17: Foods Comprising The Dash Diet

The foods we consume on a daily basis have an effect on the types of lives we lead; as the saying goes, the foods you consume can either be your medication or your poison. Generally, what you consume will have either a positive or negative effect on your health. The DASH diet, like every other diet, has a list of permitted foods as well as a list of foods that are off limits.

The DASH diet encourages the consumption of whole cereals, fruits, vegetables, and low-fat dairy products. The amount of food you consume is also a crucial aspect of the DASH diet that must be considered. The nutritional value of each consumed product is also considered. Included in the DASH diet are salmon, legumes, and poultry. You may also consume red meat, desserts, and fats in moderation. In general, the DASH diet is minimal in saturated fats and cholesterol.

Cholesterol and saturated lipids are a leading cause of health problems, particularly hypertension and obesity. Reducing them in your daily diet helps to ward off these illnesses.

Consider these ingredients that are compatible with the DASH diet.

Grains

Grains are an essential part of the DASH diet. The crucial point is that you must consume whole grains and not excessively processed grain products. Included among these cereals may be bread, rice, and even pasta.

Whole grains contain more fiber and nutrients than refined grains, making them the optimal choice for grain consumption. For instance, brown rice can be substituted for white rice, whole-wheat pasta for conventional pasta, and whole-grain bread for white bread. When you go grocery purchasing, you should seek out grains that are labeled "2 00% whole grain." You will benefit from the DASH diet if you distinguish yourself from those who consider people who consume whole grains to be out of date. The refined cereals are devoid of fiber and other nutrients. Consuming cereals devoid of nutritional value may not be of much assistance. The benefit is the nutritional content, not the name.

Grains are inherently low in fat; therefore, avoid adding butter, cream, and cheese sauces. When you spread butter or add cream to your whole cereals, the nutritional value will change, as the majority of these ingredients are high in fats.

Vegetables

Vegetables are an essential part of the DASH diet. In this diet, greens such as collards and kale are among the most beneficial foods.Tomatoes, carrots, yams, arrowroots, broccoli, and other vegetables are rich in fiber, vitamins, and minerals including potassium and magnesium.

Most people consider vegetables to be a side dish, disregarding the fact that they can constitute a satisfying and nutrient-rich main course. Consider serving an assortment of vegetables with brown rice as a complete entrée. This will enable you to consume vegetables in the recommended amounts, as opposed to consuming vegetables only as side dishes, particularly with fatty dishes that are high in cholesterol and other unhealthy fats.

The first step in developing a positive relationship with vegetables is to stop viewing them as side dishes and start viewing them as complete entrees. I trust you will make this essential adjustment.

Fresh vegetables are delicious and easily accessible. Vegetables that are frozen and labeled as low in sodium and without added additives are also healthy options.

Here are some tips to help you increase your daily vegetable intake. You can reduce your meat intake while doubling your vegetable intake. Include vegetables in every meal, but don't reinterpret this as an excuse to consume vegetables as a side dish.

Four to five servings of vegetables are beneficial to the DASH diet.

Fruits

Just like vegetables, fruits also contain vital minerals like potassium and magnesium. The fruits also contain fiber and other essential micronutrients that are essential to the body and immune system development. The majority of fruits are also minimal in fat, with the exception of avocados and coconuts. The fruits can be consumed with each meal or as a refreshment. If you want to keep your health in excellent condition, maintain a healthy weight, and reduce your risk of developing hypertension, you should replace highly processed snacks like hamburgers with fruits.

You can also make fresh fruit desserts to increase your fruit consumption. You can enjoy a slice of mango with your entrée, pawpaw as an appetizer, and a fresh fruit assortment for dessert.

The edible peels of most fruits are also beneficial because they are rich in fiber. Apple, lemon, and pear peels, as well as the peels of other fruits with pits, enhance the texture of certain recipes and are a healthier option. Lemon peels are also beneficial for throat issues and can alleviate sore throat when immersed in raw honey.

If you're taking medication, it's a good idea to confirm that eating certain fruits is safe. Certain fruits, notably citrus fruits, may interact with your medications; therefore, you should double-check with your pharmacist.

It is preferable to use fresh fruits because they are nutritionally complete and free of additives, but if you can only locate canned fruits, please verify that they do not contain added sugars. This is because fruits contain simple carbohydrates such as sucrose and fructose, which are readily absorbed into the bloodstream, as opposed to other canned fruits, which contain added complex sugars. Added carbohydrates are detrimental to hypertension because they exacerbate the condition.

Four to five servings of fruits are beneficial to the DASH diet.

Dairy Products Dairy products such as milk, yogurt, and cheese are significant sources of calcium, vitamin D, and protein. If you do not verify the fat content of the dairy product you are using, the beneficial qualities may be altered. It is recommended that you utilize low-fat or, even better, fat-free dairy products. If you do not monitor the fat content, dairy products can be a significant source of fat, which is counterproductive to your efforts to avoid hypertension.

The low-fat and fat-free dairy products are equally delicious, so you will have no trouble consuming the recommended amount. Avoid consuming fatty dairy products.

Even if the cheese is fat-free, it is still recommended to limit your consumption. This is because it typically contains a high sodium content.

Two to three servings of dairy per day are advised.

lean meat, seafood, and poultry

Meat is an exceptionally abundant source of protein, B vitamins, iron, and zinc. But it also contains fats and cholesterol, which are neither helpful for hypertension prevention nor weight loss. When cholesterol levels in the blood vessels are elevated, the blood vessels become constricted, resulting in an increase in intravascular pressure. Even lean meat contains cholesterol, so it's advisable to reduce meat consumption. Reduce your meat consumption and increase your vegetable consumption to replace the void.

When consuming poultry, it is recommended to remove the skin due to its high lipid content. The DASH diet reduces fat consumption, so fat sources should be eliminated.

Meat and poultry can also be baked, broiled, grilled, or roasted instead of fried.

Eat fish that is good for the heart, such as salmon, herring, and tuna. These varieties of fish are rich in omega-6 fatty acids, which aid in regulating total cholesterol levels.

10 or fewer servings per day is considered wholesome.

Nuts, seeds and legumes

Nuts and seeds, such as almonds, sunflower seeds, kidney beans, peas, and lentils, are excellent sources of magnesium, potassium, and protein. Nuts, seeds, and legumes are also rich in fiber and phytochemicals, which are plant compounds that aid in the prevention of certain malignancies and cardiovascular diseases. However, they should be consumed in smaller quantities due to their high caloric content.

Nuts are frequently criticized for their high fat content, but fortunately they contain healthy lipids, such as monounsaturated fat and omega-6 fatty acids. Due to their high caloric content, you should consume them sparingly.

Tofu and tempeh are excellent substitutes for meat because they contain all of the amino acids your body requires to produce a complete protein, just like meat.

Four to five portions per week are considered healthful.

lipids and oils

Fats are beneficial because they aid in vitamin absorption and strengthen the immune system. However, excessive fat increases the risk of cardiovascular disease, diabetes, and obesity. The DASH diet strives for a healthy balance by limiting total fat to no more than 27 percent of daily calories, with an emphasis on monounsaturated fats.

Saturated and trans fats are harmful to your health because they increase your blood cholesterol and risk of coronary artery disease. Reducing your consumption of meat, butter, cheese, whole milk, cream, and eggs, as well as foods prepared with lard, solid shortening, and palm and coconut oils, helps you maintain a saturated fat intake of less than 6 percent of your total daily calories.

Trans fat is commonly found in highly processed foods such as crackers, baked products, and fried foods.

If you must use margarines, examine the label to find those with the least amount of fat.

Dash Diet regimen recommends 2 to 6 servings daily.

Sweets

The DASH diet allows you to consume desserts in moderation, so you won't have to completely abstain from them.

Choose fat-free or low-fat desserts, such as sorbets, fruit ices, jelly beans, hard confectionery, graham crackers, or low-fat cookies, when eating sweets.

You can replace refined sugar with artificial sweeteners like aspartame and sucralose (Splenda), but you should use them sparingly. You should never replace them with a healthier beverage, such as low-fat milk.

You should avoid added sugar because it has no nutritional value and may hinder your weight loss efforts by increasing your caloric intake.

Five or fewer servings per week are healthy.

Alcohol and stimulants

The DASH diet does not promote alcohol consumption. This is because excessive alcohol consumption can raise blood pressure. The DASH diet recommends that males consume no more than two alcoholic beverages per day and that women consume one less than men.

The DASH diet does not, however, address caffeine consumption. Unknown are the effects of caffeine on blood pressure. However, caffeine can potentially elevate blood pressure. Therefore, if you have hypertension, you should consult your family physician for advice on this matter.

Chapter 18: The Dash Diet And Exercise

The DASH diet aims to reduce blood pressure by encouraging individuals to consume less sodium and adhere to a low-calorie meal plan. According to the diet's proponents, the plan may help individuals lower their blood pressure in approximately fourteen days.

Meal patterns on the DASH diet range from 2 ,600 to 6 ,2 00 calories per day. In addition to adhering to the diet, dieters should combine their eating practices with regular exercise – at least 6 0 minutes per day, three times per week. Although the DASH diet does not outline a specific exercise regimen, those who have combined exercise with the low-calorie meal plan have experienced significant health improvements.

Incorporating cardiovascular exercise on the majority of weekdays or strength training a few days per week can hasten weight loss and other health benefits. If you are on the DASH diet and want to lose weight (or simply be healthy), you can perform the exercises below.

BICYCLE

Begin by reclining down on the floor. Your hands are behind your head, and your complete body should be in proper alignment. Raise your legs together at least 2 2 inches off the ground. Raise the right shoulder blade off the mat and bend forward while bringing the left knee and the right elbow together.

Completely rotate your upper body so that your left knee touches your right forearm. Return to the center and repeat the steps on the opposite side. Repeat the procedure fifteen times.

Lateral Raises

Straighten your posture and slightly separate your feet. Bent your legs slightly. Hold a dumbbell in each hand with the palms facing inward. Your limbs should be positioned at your sides. Deeply inhale and steadily raise your arms to shoulder height with your arms straight. Slowly return to the initial point. Perform 2 sets of 2 2 reps.

Diagonal Front Raises

Each fist should contain a dumbbell. Stand with your feet hip-width apart.

Your limbs should be at your sides with your palms facing backwards. Slowly raise your arms up and out to the sides at the same time. Stop once your arms reach shoulder height. In front, the limbs should form a V-shape. Slowly return to the initial position. Perform two sets of ten repetitions. If you suffer from a chronic shoulder injury, you should not undertake this exercise.

Hamstring Roll

With an exercise ball, rest flat on the ground. Your ankles should rest on the uppermost portion of the exercise ball. Extend your arms and place your palms flat on the earth. Raise your body up. Permit your body to form a straight line from your ankles to your stomach. Utilize your hamstrings to pull the object towards yourself. Strive to maintain an upright and still upper body. Return the object to its initial position with care. Perform 2 0 repetitions.

Swimming or Walking

Combining the DASH diet with physical activity, such as swimming or walking, will assist you in shedding superfluous weight and maintaining a trim physique over time. Start with a simple 2 10 - minute walk at your preferred time of day and progressively increase the duration of your activity.

You can engage in 6 0 minutes of walking or swimming at once. You may also select lesser workout durations, perhaps 2 0 minutes or less. A weekly review is required. You have a total of two and a half hours per week for moderately intense activities. If you want to attain greater health benefits, gradually increase your weekly workout time to five hours.

Spinach And Berry Salad

Ingredients

- 6 tbsp balsamic vinegar
- 6 tbsp olive oil
- 2 tsp Dijon mustard
- 2 tsp honey
- *20 cups baby spinach*
- 2 cups sliced strawberries
- 2 cups blueberries
- 1 cup chopped walnuts
- ½ cup blue cheese crumbles

- Kosher salt and freshly ground pepper, to taste

Directions

1. In a large bowl, combine spinach, strawberries, and blueberries.
2. Top with walnuts and blue cheese.
3. In a small bowl, whisk together vinegar, olive oil, mustard, honey, salt, and pepper.
4. Drizzle over salad just before serving.

Cornmeal Waffles Served With Yogurt And Fruit

Number of Servings: 8

Ingredients:

- 1/7 tsp salt
- 2 Tbsp melted unsalted butter
- 4 large egg white
- 1 Tbsp canola oil
- 4 cup low fat yogurt, unsweetened
- 12 oz fresh or frozen and thawed raspberries or blueberries
- 4 Tbsp canola oil
- 1 cup yellow cornmeal

- 1 cup whole wheat or almond flour
- 2 Tbsp coconut sugar or Stevia
- 1/7 tsp baking powder
- 1/7 cup low fat milk
- 1/7 tsp baking powder

How to Prepare:

Following the manufacturer's instructions, preheat a Teflon waffle iron.

In a mixing basin, combine the flour, baking powder, salt, sugar, and cornmeal.

Combine 1 tablespoon of canola oil with the melted butter and milk in a separate receptacle.

Combine the flour mixture and milk mixture gradually until just combined. Do not over-mix. Fold the egg white into the mixture gently.

Apply the canola oil to the waffle maker.

Pour approximately one cup of batter into the waffle iron, then follow the manufacturer's simple cooking instructions. Remove the waffle from the waffle iron and cook the remaining mixture.

On top of the waffles, distribute the yogurt and scatter the berries. Serve right away.

Chicken Ragu With Mushrooms

Ingredient Checklist

- 2 cloves grated garlic
- 30 cup tomato paste
- 20 cup dry red wine
- 20teaspoon salt
- 30teaspoon crushed red pepper
- 2 tablespoon chopped fresh rosemary
- 2 pound whole-wheat ling

50 -ounce can of whole, peeled, no-salt-added San Marzano tomatoes

- 30 cup extra-virgin olive oil
- 2 medium onion, chopped

• 2 medium carrots, chopped

• 8 ounces cremini mushrooms, quartered

• 200 pounds boneless, skinless chicken thighs, trimmed and cut into 2 -inch pieces

List of things to do

Bring an ample quantity of water to a simmer.

Tomatoes and tomato juice are poured into a medium basin. Using your hands, dice the tomatoes into pieces.

Heat oil in an electric pressure cooker on Sauté mode. Add the carrots, onion, and mushrooms. Ten minutes, stirring occasionally, or until the mushrooms have released their liquid. Combine the chicken with the garlic and tomato purée. Cook, stirring occasionally, for approximately 8 minutes, or until the chicken is evenly coated and the mixture at the bottom of the pan begins to caramelize. Add the tomatoes, wine, salt, and red pepper flakes. Cook for about 2 minutes, scraping up the browned pieces, or until the liquid begins to boil. Extinguish the fire.

Close and secure the lid. For 2 0 minutes, cook at high pressure with ease. Release the pressure manually. Mix in rosemary and stir.

Cook the pasta according to the package's instructions. The pasta is served with the sauce, cheese, and parsley after being drained.

Banana Nut Pancakes

Ingredients

- 2 cup fat-free milk
- 6 large egg whites
- 4 tsp oil
- 2 tsp vanilla
- 4 tbsp. chopped walnuts 2 cup whole wheat flour
- 4 tsp baking powder
- 1/2 tsp salt
- 1/2 tsp cinnamon
- 2 large banana, mashed

•

Instructions

Mix all dry ingredients in a large bowl

Combine milk, egg white, oil, vanilla and mashed bananas in another bowl and mix until smooth

Combine wet ingredients with the dry and mix well

Heat a large skillet on medium heat

Pour 1/2 cup of pancake batter onto warm griddle for each pancake

Breakfast Banana Split

Ingredients

- 1 cup low fat vanilla yogurt
- 1 cup canned pineapple tidbits
- 2 small banana
- 1 cup granola cereal

Instructions

1. Peel and split banana lengthwise.
2. Place half in two separate cereal bowls
3. Sprinkle granola over banana, reserving some for topping
4. Spoon yogurt on top
5. Decorate with reserved granola and pineapple before serving

Asparagus and Onion Frittata

Ingredients:

- 1 cup and 2 tablespoon of parmesan cheese, grated
- 12 large eggs
- Fresh ground pepper
- 1 teaspoon of kosher salt
- 2 medium onion, sliced thinly
- 2 teaspoon of olive oil
- 4 cups of asparagus, cut into 2 -inch pieces
- 4 teaspoons of balsamic vinegar
- 1 cup of fresh basil, sliced thinly
- 6 green onions, sliced

Directions:

1. Set the broiler to high and preheat.
2. Set a 1-5-inch ovenproof skillet over medium heat.
3. Add the olive oil.
4. Once hot, add in the onions and easy cook for 5-10 minutes.
5. Stir in the balsamic vinegar. Add 4 tablespoons of water and the asparagus.
6. Cover with a lid and steam for 5-10 minutes.
7. Whisk the eggs and add in ½ cup of the grated parmesan.

8. Mix together until well-combined and season with ½ teaspoon of kosher salt and freshly ground pepper.

9. Remove the lid from the skillet and add in the remaining kosher salt, basil, and green onions. Mix well.

10. Pour in the egg mixture into the skillet and stir briefly.

11. Easy cook for 1-5 minutes.

12. Place the skillet in the broiler and easy cook for 5-10 minutes.

13. Once done, remove the skillet from the broiler and sprinkle the remaining parmesan on top. Rest for 5-10 minutes.

14. Slice the frittata into 5-10 and serve immediately.

Berry Morning Blast

Ingredients:

- 2 cup of low fat plain yogurt
- 2 cup of rinsed blueberries
- 2 cup of low fat granola
- 2 cup of rinsed strawberries, sliced

Directions:

1. Prepare 5-10 small glasses.

2. Divide the strawberries equally between the 5-10 glasses. Sprinkle granola on top of the strawberries.

3. Divide the blueberries equally between the 5-10 glasses and place on top of the granola.

4. Spoon the yogurt on top of the blueberries and serve.

Dash Morning Quinoa

Ingredients:

½ cup honey (brown sugar will do)

4 cups quinoa (uncooked)

6 cups low-fat milk

1 cup currants (dried)

1 cup almonds (slivered or sliced)

½ tsp. cinnamon

Directions:

1. Rinse the quinoa with mineral water.
2. In a medium saucepan, bring the low-fat milk to a boil.
3. Simmer until the liquid is absorbed.
4. Cover, reduce the heat and boil for 35 to 40 minutes.
5. Remove from heat and fluff the milk using a fork.
6. Add the remaining ingredients, cover and easy cook for another 20 minutes.
7. Add the quinoa before serving.

Summer Quinoa Bowls

Ingredients:

½ tsp. vanilla extract

¼ cups low-fat milk

½ cup quinoa (rinsed and cooked)

2 peach (sliced)

6 tsp. honey

30 blueberries

20 raspberries

6 tsp. brown sugar

Directions:

1. Combine brown sugar, vanilla and 1/2 cup of milk in a saucepan.
2. Easy cook under medium-high heat for 25 to 30 minutes.
3. Reduce heat to low, cover and easy cook for another 25 to 30 minutes or until a fluff forms.
4. In a grill pan meanwhile, spray a small amount of cooking oil. Add the peaches and easy cook for 5-10 minutes.
5. Remove the milk and vanilla mixture from heat.
6. Transfer the mixture into a medium bowl and microwave for 1-5 minutes.
7. Divide the cooked quinoa into 6 bowls.

8. Pour in the milk and top it with blueberries, raspberries and the remaining peaches.
9. Drizzle each bowl with a teaspoon of honey and serve.

Spiced Salmon

Ingredients

- 1 teaspoon pepper
- 1/2 teaspoon dill weed
- Dash salt
- Dash dried tarragon
- Dash cayenne pepper
- 2 salmon fillet (2 pounds)
- 4 tablespoons packed brown sugar
- 2 tablespoon soy sauce
- 2 tablespoon butter, melted
- 2 tablespoon olive oil
- 1 teaspoon garlic powder

- 1 teaspoon ground mustard
- 1 teaspoon paprika

Directions

1. Mix all ingredients except salmon; brush over salmon.
2. Place salmon, skin side down, on an oiled grill rack or on a lightly oiled baking sheet.
3. Grill, covered, over medium heat or broil 5-10 in.
4. from heat until fish just begins to flake easily with a fork, 25 to 30 minutes.

Tomato Vegetable Soup

Ingredients

- 2 garlic clove, minced
- 6 cups diced fresh tomatoes
- 1/2 cup minced fresh basil or 2 tablespoon dried basil
- 1 teaspoon salt
- 1/2 teaspoon pepper
- 2 cup chopped onion
- 2 cup chopped carrots
- 4 teaspoons butter
- 12 cups reduced-sodium chicken or vegetable broth
- 2 pound fresh green beans, cut into 2 -inch pieces

Directions

1. In a large saucepan, saute onion and carrots in butter for 5-10 minutes.
2. Stir in the broth, beans and garlic; bring to a boil.
3. Reduce heat; cover and simmer for 35 to 40 minutes or until vegetables are tender.
4. Stir in the tomatoes, basil, salt and pepper.
5. Cover and simmer 5-10 minutes longer.

Spaghetti Squash Dash

Ingredients:

- 2 8 1 ounces tomatoes, diced;
- 4 cloves of garlic, chopped;
- 4 tablespoons of tomato paste;
- 16 ounces tomato sauce;
- A 6 -pound spaghetti squash, cooked; and
- Small basil leaves.
- 2 1 teaspoons of dried Italian seasoning, crushed;
- 2 pound of lean, ground beef;
- 1/7 teaspoon of black peppers;
- 1 cup green pepper, chopped;
- 1 cup onion, chopped;
- ½ cup of Parmesan cheese; shredded;

Instructions:

1. In a skillet, easy cook together the garlic, pepper, onion, and ground beef until the ground beef becomes brown.

2. Add the drained diced tomatoes, tomato sauce, tomato paste, Italian seasoning, and black pepper into the skillet.

3. When the mixture starts to boil, bring down the heat and let the spaghetti sauce mixture simmer for up to 25 to 30 minutes.

4. While letting the sauce simmer, prick your spaghetti squash microwave in a microwave-safe dish for 25 to 30 minutes or when it turns tender.

5. When done, allow the squash to stand for up to 5-10 minutes before removing its seeds, shredding it, and separating it's pulp to form strands or noodles.

6. Slather the squash noodles with the spaghetti sauce and enjoy!

6 . Baked Oatmeal

8.
Ingredients:

- 6 cups rolled oats (uncooked)
- 4 tsp baking powder
- 2 tsp cinnamon
- 2 cup skim milk
- 2 tbsp canola oil
- 1 cup unsweetened applesauce
- 1/2 cup brown sugar
- Egg substitute equivalent to 2 eggs, or 8 egg whites

Directions:

1. Preheat oven to 350°F (150 °C).
2. In a medium bowl, lightly beat the eggs and sugar, then whisk in the oil and applesauce.
3. Add the oats, cinnamon, baking powder and milk and mix well to combine.
4. Generously oil a 9x13 baking dish with cooking spray.
5. Pour the oatmeal mixture into the prepared baking dish and bake in the oven for 6 o minutes until set and lightly golden.

Shrimp Salad With Avocado

Ingredients:

- 1/2 cup red onion (chopped)
- 4 limes juice
- 2 tsp olive oil
- 2 tbsp cilantro (chopped)
- Pinch of salt and fresh pepper
- 2 lb (8 10 0 g) jumbo cooked shrimp (peeled and deveined, chopped)
- 2 medium tomato (diced)
- 2 avocado (diced)

- 2 jalapeno (seeds removed, finely diced)

Directions:

1. Place red onion, olive oil, and lime juice in a small bowl, season with salt and pepper.
2. Let stand for at least 5-10 minutes to mix flavors.
3. Now place together avocado, jalapeño, chopped shrimp and tomato in a large salad bowl.
4. Spoon the marinade mixture over the shrimp mixture, sprinkle with chopped cilantro and mix to combine.
5. Place the salad in a serving plate and enjoy.

Savory Yogurt Bowls

Ingredients:

- 2 tsp. dried oregano
- 1/2 tsp. freshly ground black pepper
- 4 c. nonfat plain Greek yogurt
- 1 c. slivered almonds
- 2 medium cucumber, diced
- 1 c. pitted Kalamata olives, halved
- 4 tbsp. fresh lemon juice
- 2 tbsp. extra-virgin olive oil

Directions:

1. In a small bowl, mix the cucumber, olives, lemon juice, oil, oregano, and pepper.
2. Divide the yogurt evenly among 5-10 storage containers.
3. Top with the cucumber-olive mix and almonds.

www.ingramcontent.com/pod-product-compliance
Lightning Source LLC
Chambersburg PA
CBHW060459030426
42337CB00015B/1646